Herbal Antibiotics Power

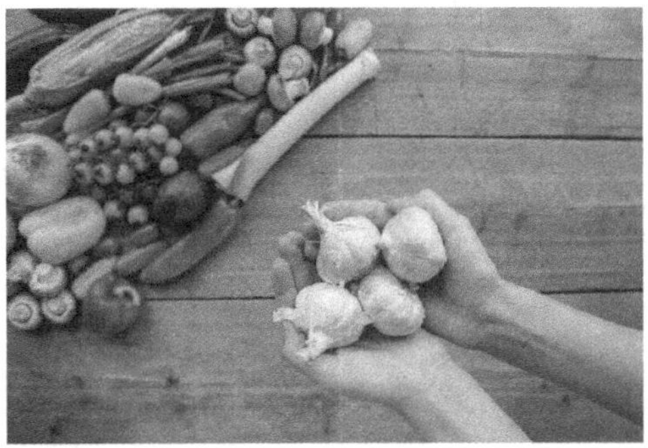

Harnessing the Arsenal for Optimal wellness

2024

By

Clark Tyler

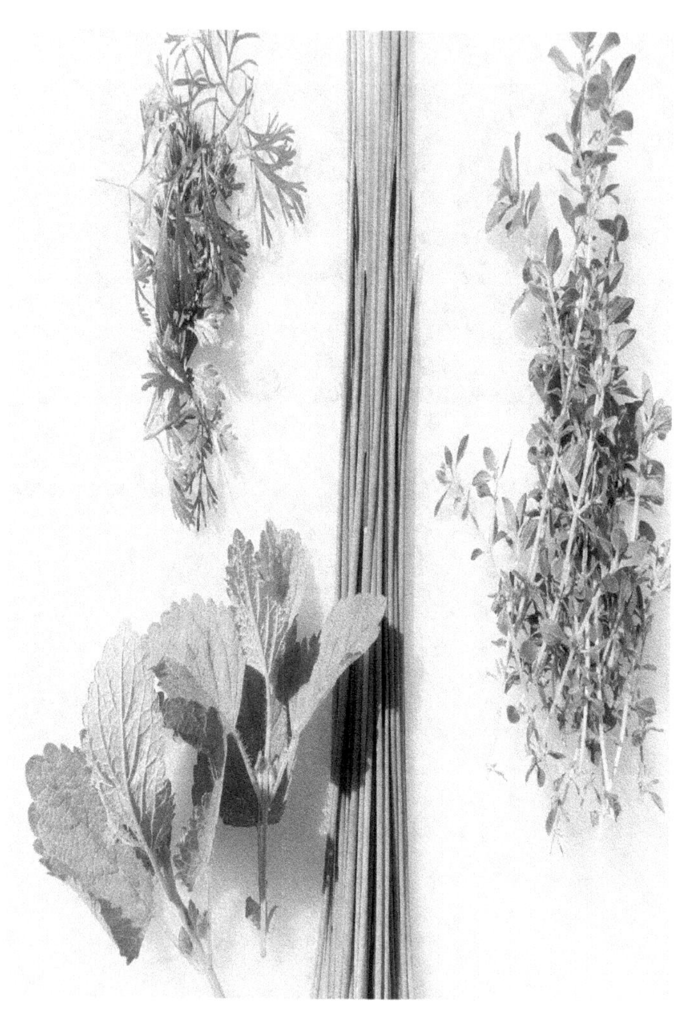

Table of Contents

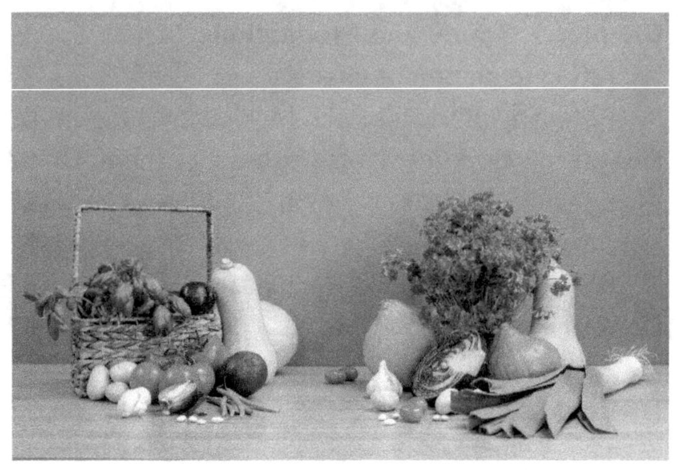

Introduction

Brief Overview of Herbal Antibiotics

Natural antibiotics are not the only options available to us; herbal antibiotics, with their inherent healing qualities, offer a strong substitute for conventional antibiotics. Among the many people who are becoming more skeptical of artificial remedies, these plant protectors show great promise for preserving human health. Imagine the strong aroma of garlic, which is not only a culinary wonder but also a powerful source of allicin, a bioactive substance with strong antibacterial properties. Research has shown that it can fight off several kinds of illnesses and provide a natural defense against them. Garlic, a culinary staple with a heady aroma, contains carvacrol, a powerful antibacterial that goes after bacteria at their base. In the world of herbs, echinacea is a colorful blossom that shows off echinacea, a substance that is thought to strengthen the immune system. As we explore the world of herbal antibiotics, it's important to acknowledge their potential advantages—not as stand-ins but as friends in the quest for a strong constitution. Their effectiveness is not the only thing that makes them appealing; there is also a decreased chance of side effects, which are common with synthetic antibiotics. These medicines seem to have been carefully balanced by nature, in its wisdom, to meet the complex demands of the human system.Natural antibiotics are not the only options available to us; herbal antibiotics, with their inherent healing qualities, offer a strong substitute for conventional antibiotics. Among the many people who are becoming more skeptical of artificial remedies, these plant protectors show great promise for preserving human health. Imagine the strong aroma of garlic, which is not only a culinary wonder but also a powerful source of allicin, a bioactive substance with strong antibacterial properties. Research has shown that it can fight off several kinds of illnesses and provide a natural defense against them. Garlic, a culinary staple with a heady aroma, contains carvacrol, a powerful antibacterial that goes after bacteria at their base. In the world of herbs, echinacea is a colorful blossom that shows off echinacea, a substance that is thought to strengthen the immune system. As we explore the world of herbal antibiotics, it's important to acknowledge their potential advantages—not as stand-ins but as friends in the quest for a strong constitution. Their effectiveness is not the only thing that makes them appealing; there is also a decreased chance of side effects, which are common with synthetic antibiotics. These medicines seem to have been carefully balanced by nature, in its wisdom, to meet the complex demands of the human system.

But proceed with caution along this lush trail. The lack of scientific agreement on herbal antibiotics and the potential for adverse reactions or combinations with prescription drugs highlight the need for making well-informed judgments. It is crucial to speak with a healthcare professional before adopting these plant-powered warriors to ensure that herbal medicine and traditional medical treatment work in concert. Herbal antibiotics play a seductive note in this symphony of health, beckoning inquiry into the wide-ranging field where human health and nature's medicine collide. These plant partners beckon, providing a complex and engrossing way to support our bodies in the continuous drama of health and healing, even as science works to unlock their mysteries.

Importance of Optimal wellness

Humans value optimal wellbeing for a variety of reasons that affect many aspects of life. To begin with, it strengthens the immune system, which serves as a barrier against diseases and infections. The body can efficiently fight off illnesses when it is in optimal health, which lowers the frequency and severity of ailments. Additionally, mental clarity and cognitive performance are critically dependent on overall wellbeing. A healthy lifestyle that includes regular exercise, a balanced diet, and enough sleep has a good impact on brain health. As a result, memory, focus, and general cognitive function are all enhanced. Achieving both personal and professional objectives, as well as improving productivity and decision-making, depend on this kind of mental health. Another essential component of ideal well-being is emotional resilience. People who are in strong mental health are more resilient to stress and hardship. They develop coping strategies, sustain steady connections, and demonstrate emotional intelligence. This enhances pleasure on an individual level and has a good knock-on effect on families, companies, and communities. Moreover, lifespan and quality of life are linked to good wellbeing. People who develop healthy behaviors are more likely to live longer, more active lives. In addition to helping people directly, this lessens the strain on healthcare systems and promotes a more long-term approach to public health. Social cohesion and a sense of belonging are fostered by excellent well-being. People in good health are more likely to participate in social activities and have strong support systems. This sense of social cohesiveness fosters general wellbeing and fosters an atmosphere that is conducive to personal development and fulfillment. A population that prioritizes optimal wellbeing can result in lower healthcare expenditures and more productivity from an economic standpoint. Healthy people are more likely to participate fully in the workforce, which reduces healthcare costs and absenteeism. The significance of achieving optimal wellbeing essentially rests in its all-encompassing influence on lifespan, mental health, emotional stability, physical health, social dynamics, and economic vigor. It is a comprehensive strategy that improves people's lives on a personal level and has a beneficial ripple impact on entire economies and civilizations.

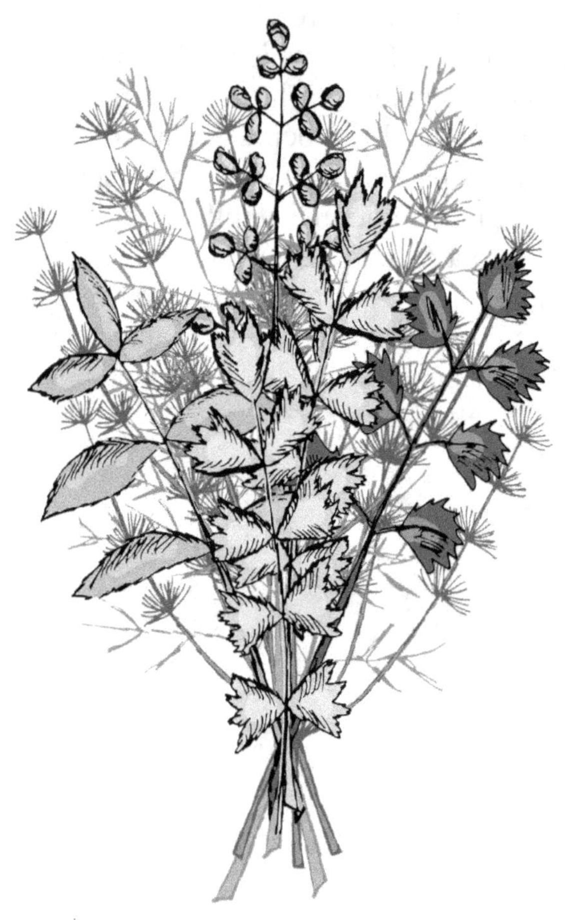

Chapter 1: Understanding Herbal Antibiotics

Definition of Herbal Antibiotics

Herbal antibiotics are substances derived from plants that possess antimicrobial qualities, meaning they can either combat or impede the growth of germs. Many times, these natural substitutes are thought to possess therapeutic qualities akin to those of conventional antibiotics, providing possible advantages without the artificial substances included in conventional drugs. It's crucial to remember that there is conflicting scientific data on the safety and effectiveness of herbal antibiotics, so speaking with a healthcare provider is advised before using them exclusively to treat serious illnesses.

A knowledgeable healer by the name of Elara once learned of the amazing healing properties concealed inside the world of herbs in a little town tucked away between beautiful forests and rolling hills. Elara set out to discover the secrets of nature when the community was plagued by an enigmatic sickness that defied medical diagnosis.

She learned about plants with strong antibacterial qualities by poring over old books and talking to the town herbalist. Through her quest, Elara found a hidden gem of natural substances hidden in the forest's verdant fabric: herbal antibiotics.

She happened found a unique plant called "Verdant Guardian" one day. There were whispers in legend that this plant was the secret to curing the hardest-to-treat illnesses. Elara carefully combined the essence of several plants to create a powerful elixir.

The previously sick town saw a miraculous reversal as the residents enthusiastically embraced this natural treatment. Their mystery disease started to fade, and they became healthy and energetic again.

Elara clarified that herbal antibiotics were nature's defense mechanisms against microbial intruders. Garlic brandished its powerful sword of allicin, echinacea served as a watchful shield, and oregano oil appeared as a cunning assassin against pathogenic microorganisms. With its origins in gold, goldenseal acted as a protector, bolstering the body's defenses.

The story of Elara and her natural antibiotics went viral, serving as a ray of hope for many looking for alternatives to traditional medication. Elara had discovered a deeper link in the complex dance between nature and humans—a comprehensive solution based on rational harmony with the surroundings.

Thus, the hamlet not only recovered but flourished, with the legacy of herbal antibiotics continuing to work its curative magic throughout successive generations, serving as a constant reminder that sometimes the best remedies lie in the verdant embrace of nature.

Types of Herbal Antibiotics

1. Allium sativum, or garlic: Allicin, a strong antibacterial substance, is found in garlic. By rupturing bacterial cell membranes, allicin prevents bacteria from growing. It's a natural antibiotic that works well against a variety of germs. For instance, allicin from garlic showed antibacterial action against common pathogens, such as Staphylococcus aureus and E. coli, in research.

2. Echinacea:Echinacea purpurea Echinacea boosts white blood cell formation through immune system stimulation. Respiratory infections are lessened and prevented in part by its antibacterial properties. For instance,

echinacea extracts have demonstrated effectiveness in lessening the intensity and length of respiratory tract infections, demonstrating the plant's immune-stimulating and antimicrobial qualities.

3. Hydrastis canadensis, or goldenseal: Berberine, a substance with broad-spectrum antibacterial effects, is found in goldenseal. Berberine lowers inflammation and interferes with the operation of bacterial cells. For instance, the efficacy of berberine found in goldenseal against a variety of bacteria, including those that cause gastrointestinal infections, has been investigated.

4. Origanum vulgare (oregano): Carvacrol-rich oregano oil has strong antimicrobial qualities. Carvacrol breaks down the cell membranes of bacteria to prevent them from growing. For instance, oregano oil's potential as a natural antibiotic has been demonstrated by its ability to display antibacterial activity against a variety of strains.

5. Turmeric (Curcuma longa):The compound curcumin has anti-inflammatory and antibacterial qualities. It facilitates healing and aids in immune response modulation. Example: Studies have shown that curcumin has antibacterial properties against a range of

microorganisms, making it a useful herbal medicine.

6. Zingiber officinale (ginger): Compounds such as gingerol are responsible for the antibacterial effects of ginger. It reduces inflammation and aids in the fight against infections. For instance, ginger has long been used to cure illnesses, and studies on extracts from the plant have demonstrated antibacterial efficacy against pathogens.

7. Thyme (Thymus vulgaris): Thyme has a strong antibacterial component called thymol. Thymol is useful in treating cutaneous and respiratory infections because it breaks down bacterial cell membranes. For instance, thymol in thyme oil has proven to be effective against a variety of bacterial strains, indicating its potential use as a natural antibiotic.

8. (Azadirachta indica, or neem): Justification: Neem is a plant that has several antibacterial components. It is used for immunological support, dental care, and skin disorders. It inhibits the growth of microorganisms.

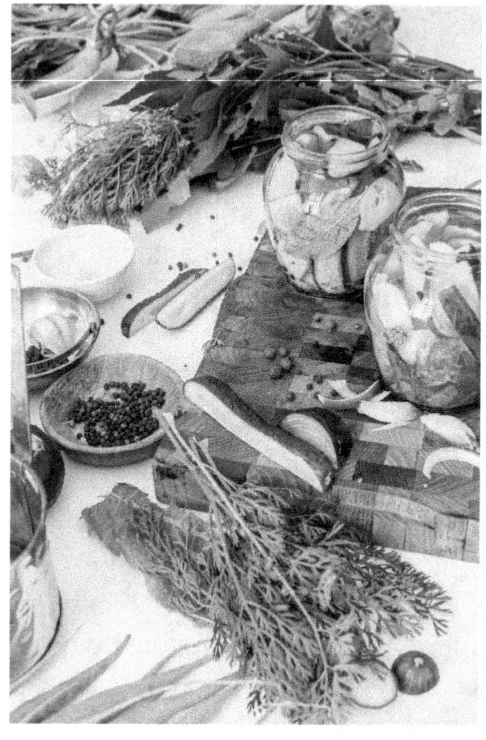

For instance, the antibacterial activity of neem extracts against common pathogens highlights the plant's use in traditional medicine for infections.

Historical uses and cultural significance of Herbal Antibiotics

Traditional medicine has a long history of using herbal antibiotics, which are made from a wide range of plants that have been used medicinally by tribes all over the world. Herbal antibiotics have been used historically for thousands of years; ancient Egyptian, Greek, and Chinese cultures all used a variety of plants in their medicinal regimens. Because of their antibacterial qualities, therapeutic herbs like aloe vera and garlic were used in ancient Egypt. Papyrus scrolls with records of these treatments demonstrate a highly developed knowledge of herbal medicine. The Egyptians' expertise was passed down to the Greeks, who increased the use of plants in medicine. Hippocrates, who is frequently seen as the founder of Western medicine, recommended the use of antimicrobial plants like oregano and thyme. Herbs such as licorice root and astragalus were prized in traditional Chinese medicine, which took a holistic approach to healing, for their capacity to bolster the body's indigenous defenses. Compiling over many years, the Chinese herbal pharmacopeia displays the complex understanding of employing plants to treat illnesses. Herbal antibiotics were extremely important for treating a wide range of illnesses in Europe throughout the Middle Ages. Local plants were vital to populations that had limited access to advanced medical services. Due to its antibacterial qualities, garlic was a common ingredient in many medieval medicines. Herbs like echinacea and yarrow were also frequently used in traditional medicine. Globally, traditional medical practices have made extensive use of herbal antibiotics. For example, Native American cultures used herbs with antibacterial properties, such as echinacea and goldenseal. These customs, which have been passed down through the years, represent a close relationship between natural treatments and culture. Herbal antibiotics became less common in many Western civilizations in the 20th century as pharmaceutical antibiotics were more widely used. Nonetheless, there has been a renaissance of interest in traditional medicine in recent years as scientists look at the scientific underpinnings of the effectiveness of certain plants. Concerns about antibiotic resistance and a desire for more environmentally friendly and natural healthcare options are what are driving this comeback. Herbal antibiotics are still widely used in culture, serving as both medicines and markers of a people's identity and kinship with the natural world. Their historical applications highlight the timeless wisdom of traditional therapeutic methods, bridging the gap between the past and present in the pursuit of holistic well-being.

Differentiating from pharmaceutical antibiotics

Herbal and pharmaceutical antibiotiantibioticscs are two different strategies for treating bacterial infections, each having special traits and issues to take into account. Pharmaceutical are artificial substances made by chemical reactions that are designed to attack particular bacterial defense systems. Penicillin, for example, prevents bacteria from synthesizing their cell walls, whereas ciprofloxacin prevents DNA replication. These medications are put through rigorous testing in regulated settings to guarantee uniform doses, safety, and effectiveness. The FDA and other regulatory bodies supervise and authorize these drugs. On the other hand, herbal antibiotics use the antibacterial properties found in plants. One such example is garlic, which has antibacterial qualities due to the presence of allicin. However, because plant composition varies naturally, consistent doses are rarely seen in herbal treatments. Herbal antibiotics are subject to less strict regulatory scrutiny than pharmaceuticals, which leads to a wider variety of products with differing degrees of safety and efficacy.

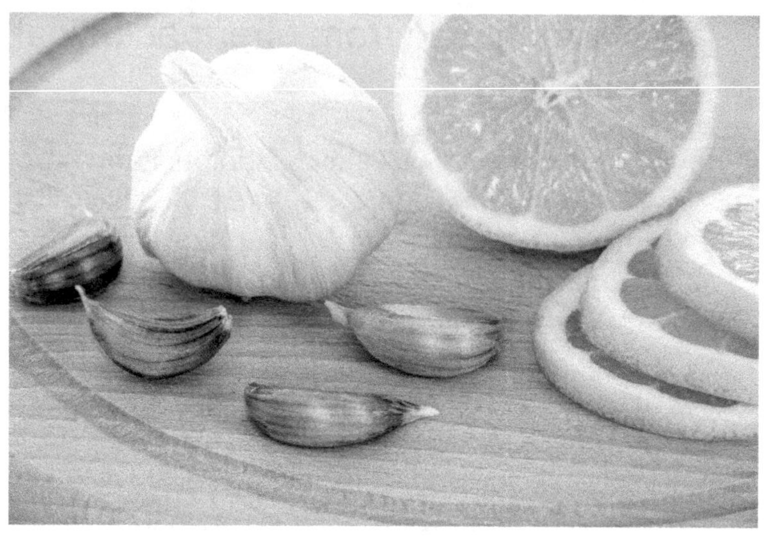

Pharmaceutical antibiotics have defined administration methods and provide accuracy and consistency. On the other hand, the potency and purity of herbal antibiotics might vary depending on other factors, such as the circumstances of plant production. Herbal alternatives may not have undergone as thorough an investigation as pharmaceutical antibiotics, which leaves gaps in our knowledge of their efficacy and possible adverse effects. The decision between pharmaceutical and herbal antibiotics is influenced by a number of variables, including the degree of the illness, personal health preferences, and the need for therapies based on solid scientific data.

Chapter Two: The Arsenal of Herbal Antibiotics

Highlighting Potent Herbs

Of course! This is a brief synopsis of 30 strong herbs and their advantages:

1. Turmeric (Curcuma longa): promotes joint health, is an antioxidant, and reduces inflammation.

2. Ginger (Zingiber officinale): promotes healthy digestion, reduces nausea, and reduces inflammation.

3. Garlic (Allium sativum) supports the cardiovascular system and the immune system.

4. Cinnamon (Cinnamomum verum): anti-inflammatory and blood sugar regulator.

5. Peppermint (Mentha × piperita): reduces headaches and facilitates digestion.

6. Chamomile (Matricaria chamomilla): relaxing, anti-inflammatory, and sleep-promoting.

7. Lavender (Lavandula angustifolia): reduces stress and encourages rest.

8. Echinacea: immune system support
(Echinacea purpurea).

9. Ginseng (Panax ginseng): an adaptogen that
increases vitality and mental acuity. 10.
Withania somnifera, or ashwagandha:
adaptogenic, calming, and energizing.

11. Milk thistle (Silybum marianum): promotes
detoxification and liver health.

12. Holy Basil (Ocimum sanctum):
anti-inflammatory, adaptogen, and stress
reliever.

13. Nettle (Urtica dioica): anti-inflammatory
and high in vitamins and minerals.

14. Rosemary (Rosmarinus officinalis):
antioxidant and memory booster.

15. Astragalus: immune support and anti-aging
properties (Astragalus membranaceus).

16. Glycyrrhiza glabra, or licorice root, reduces
inflammation and soothes gastrointestinal
problems.

17Fennel (Foeniculum vulgare): Promotes
healthy digestion and reduces inflammation.

18. Dandelions (Taraxacum officinale): diuretic
and liver-supporting.

19. Sage (Salvia officinalis): anti-inflammatory, cognitive function.

20. Origanum vulgare, or oregano: antibacterial and anti-inflammatory

21. Thyme (Thymus vulgaris): promotes respiratory health and has antimicrobial properties.

22. Actaea racemosa, or black cohosh, relieves menopausal symptoms.

23. Valerian root (Valeriana officinalis): relaxing, promotes slumber.

24. Ginkgo Biloba: Enhances memory and cognitive function.

25. Hypericum perforatum, or St. John's Wort: mild antidepressant, mood support.

26. Hawthorn (Crataegus monogyna): Support for the cardiovascular system.

27. Saw palmetto (Serenoa repens): anti-inflammatory, prostate health.

28. Vaccinium myrtillus, or bilberry: antioxidant, eye health.

29. Evening primrose (Oenothera biennis): skin health and hormone balance.

30. Passionflower (Passiflora incarnata): lessens anxiety, promotes sleep, and is calming.

It's crucial to remember that while these herbs may have a variety of health advantages, each person may respond differently, so it's best to speak with a healthcare provider before using them regularly—especially if you have any underlying medical issues or are already on medication.

Examining the medicinal properties

Of course! The thirty herbs that were previously discussed have a variety of therapeutic qualities that contribute to their standing as effective natural treatments.

1. Curcuma longa, or turmeric: Turmeric, which is well-known for its main ingredient, curcumin, has strong anti-inflammatory and antioxidant qualities that make it useful for treating illnesses like arthritis and boosting immune system function in general.

2. Zingiber officinale, or ginger: Ginger relieves nausea and inflammation, improves digestion, lessens motion sickness, and may lessen pain in the muscles.

3. Allium sativum, or garlic: Garlic is well known for strengthening the immune system and supporting the cardiovascular system, which includes lowering cholesterol and blood pressure.

4. Cinnamomum verum, or cinnamon: In addition to its taste, cinnamon has anti-inflammatory and blood sugar-regulating qualities that may help people with diabetes.

5. Mentha × piperita, or peppermint: The calming properties of peppermint also help with digestion, indigestion, and tension headaches.

6. Matricaria chamomilla, or chamomile: Well-known for its relaxing qualities, chamomile also has anti-inflammatory and sleep-inducing qualities.

7. Lavandula angustifolia, or lavender: In addition to having a nice scent, lavender is known to relieve tension, encourage relaxation, and facilitate sleep.

8. Echinacea, often known as Echinacea purpurea: Echinacea, a popular immune system booster, may lessen the intensity and length of colds.

9. Panax ginseng, or ginseng: Ginseng is an adaptogen that improves energy and mental

clarity by assisting the body in adjusting to stress.

10. Withania somnifera, or ashwagandha: Ashwagandha, another adaptogenic plant, promotes energy, well-being, and the reduction of stress.

These plants, which include nettle, holy basil, and milk thistle, have a number of health advantages. While holy basil serves as an adaptogen and an anti-inflammatory, milk thistle supports liver function and detoxification.

Nettle is prized for its anti-inflammatory qualities and is high in vitamins and minerals. Astragalus, licorice root, and rosemary help the immune system, provide digestive comfort, and enhance cognitive function, respectively.

Sage has advantages for cognitive function, while dandelion and fennel promote liver health and digestion.

Black cohosh, thyme, and oregano all have antibacterial, respiratory support, and menopausal symptom-relieving qualities. Valerian promotes rest and sleep, and ginkgo biloba improves mental clarity.

Saw palmetto, hawthorn, and St. John's Wort, in that order, have qualities that promote prostate health, improve mood, and improve cardiovascular health.

Passionflower helps with relaxation and sleep; bilberry supports eye health; and evening primrose supports skin and hormone balance. Individual reactions may differ, but integrating these herbs into a well-rounded lifestyle may offer comprehensive health advantages.

It is best to speak with medical specialists before using it, especially if you are on medication or have a pre-existing ailment.

Preparation Guidelines

1. Turmeric (Curcuma longa): Boil water to make turmeric tea. Add one teaspoon of freshly grated or powdered turmeric. Simmer for ten minutes. If desired, strain and add honey or lemon.

2. Zingiber officinale, or ginger: To make ginger tea, finely chop or shred fresh ginger. For five to ten minutes, soak ginger in boiling water. If desired, strain and add honey or lemon. As an alternative, include fresh ginger in food.

3. Garlic (Allium sativum): Use it in stir-fries, sauces, or soups. Crush or chop it before cooking.

4. Cinnamon (Cinnamomum verum): To make cinnamon tea, mix one teaspoon of ground cinnamon or a cinnamon stick with a cup of boiling water. For ten minutes, steep. If desired, strain and sweeten.

5. Peppermint (Mentha × piperita): Use dried or fresh leaves to make peppermint tea. Soak for five to ten minutes in hot water. If desired, strain and sweeten.

6. Chamomile (Matricaria chamomilla): Steep dried chamomile flowers in boiling water for five to ten minutes in order to make chamomile tea. If desired, strain and add honey or lemon.

7. Lavender (Lavandula angustifolia): Use dried lavender blossoms to make lavender tea. Take 5-7 minutes to steep in boiling water. If desired, strain and sweeten. Add oil to infuse for cooking.

8. Echinacea (Echinacea purpurea): Use dried leaves and blossoms to prepare echinacea tea. Soak for ten to fifteen minutes in hot water. If desired, strain and sweeten.

9. Ginseng (Panax ginseng): Use ginseng slices or powder while making ginseng tea. For fifteen minutes, steep in boiling water. If desired, add honey after straining.

10. Ashwagandha (Withania somnifera): Use ashwagandha root powder to make ashwagandha tea. Add a teaspoon to heated milk and sweeten to taste.

11. Milk Thistle (Silybum marianum): Crush the seeds to make milk thistle tea. Let it steep for ten minutes in boiling water. If desired, strain and sweeten.

12. Holy Basil (Ocimum sanctum): Use fresh or dried leaves to make holy basil tea. Take 5-7 minutes to steep in boiling water. If desired, strain and sweeten.

13. Nettle (Urtica dioica): Use dried nettle leaves to make nettle tea. Soak for five to ten minutes in hot water. If desired, strain and sweeten.

14. Rosemary (Rosmarinus officinalis): Use dried or fresh rosemary while making rosemary tea. Let it steep for ten minutes in boiling water. If desired, strain and sweeten.

15. Astragalus (Astragalus membranaceus): Use dried astragalus root slices to prepare astragalus

tea. Give it a 15–20 minute simmer in water. If desired, strain and sweeten.

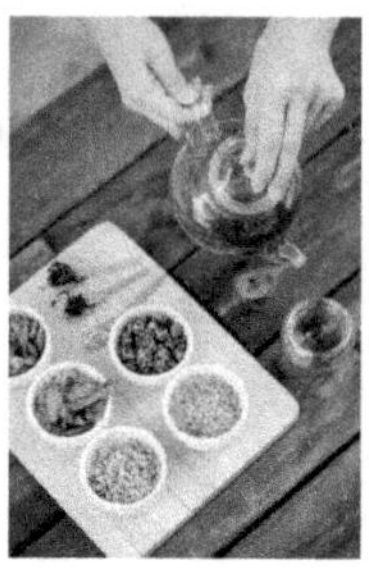

Of course! This is the next section of the detailed recipe for the following fifteen herbs to prepare:

16. Glycyrrhiza glabra, or licorice root: preparation: use dried licorice root to make licorice root tea. Soak in warm water for five to seven minutes. - Strain and add sugar, if preferred.

17. Foeniculum vulgare, or fennel: Readiness: Crush the fennel seeds to make fennel tea. Soak in warm water for ten minutes. - Strain, and if desired, add honey. As an alternative, add fennel to your food.

18. Taraxacum officinale, or dandelion: Readiness: Use dried dandelion roots to make dandelion root tea. Boil for ten to fifteen

minutes in water. - Strain and add sugar, if preferred. In salads, use fresh leaves.

19. Salvia officinalis, or sage: Readiness: Use dried or fresh sage leaves to make sage tea. Soak in warm water for five to seven minutes. Strain and add sugar, if preferred. Incorporate sage into recipes.

20. Origanum vulgare, or oregano: Readiness: Use dried or fresh oregano for your oregano tea. Soak in warm water for ten minutes. - Strain and add sugar, if preferred. When cooking, add the oregano. Thyme (Thymus vulgaris):

21. Readiness: Use dried or fresh thyme to make thyme tea. Soak in warm water for five to seven minutes. Strain and add sugar, if preferred. Include thyme in the recipe.

22. Actaea racemosa, or black cohosh: Readiness: Use black cohosh root to make black cohosh tea. Steep for ten to fifteen minutes in boiling water. - Strain and add sugar, if preferred.

23. Valerian (Valeriana officinalis) Readiness:Use dried valerian roots to make valerian tea. Steep for ten to fifteen minutes in boiling water. - Strain and add sugar, if preferred. Use with caution.

24: Ginkgo Biloba: Readiness: Follow the manufacturer's instructions while using Ginkgo Biloba supplements.

25. Hypericum perforatum, or St. John's Wort: Preparation: Take St. John's Wort supplements or extracts as recommended by the manufacturer.

26. Crataegus monogyna, or hawthorn: Readiness: Use dried hawthorn berries to make hawthorn tea. Soak in warm water for ten minutes. - Strain and add sugar, if preferred. Use with caution.

27. Serenoa repens, or saw palmetto: Readiness: Eat saw palmetto supplements in accordance with the manufacturer's instructions.

28. Vaccinium myrtillus, or bilberry: Readiness: Savor fresh bilberries or take bilberry supplements according to the manufacturer's instructions.

29. Oenothera biennis, or Evening Primrose: Setting Up: Take supplements containing evening primrose oil as recommended by the manufacturer.

30. Passiflora incarnata, or passionflower: Readiness: Use dried passionflower blooms and leaves to make passionflower tea. Soak in warm

water for ten minutes. - Strain and add sugar, if preferred. Use with caution.

Recall that these preparations are only suggestions. Before taking any herbs, especially as supplements, speak with a medical expert to be sure they are safe and helpful for your particular requirements.

Herbal dosages can differ depending on a number of things, including the person's health, any pre-existing medical issues, and the herb's form (tea, pills, etc.). Seeking individualized guidance from a healthcare practitioner is essential. For some of the plants indicated, nevertheless, the following basic guidelines apply, taking into account typical adult dosages:

Regarding Adults:

1. 500–2,000 mg of curcumin per day from turmeric (Curcuma longa).

2. Zingiber officinale (ginger): Consume up to 4 grams of ginger daily.

3. 600–1,200 mg of garlic extract daily (Allium sativum).

4. 500–2,500 mg of cinnamon (Cinnamomum verum) daily.

5. Cinnamon (Mentha × piperita): Drink one to two cups of peppermint tea daily.

6. Matricaria chamomilla (chamomile): Drink one to two glasses of chamomile tea daily.

7. Lavender (Lavandula angustifolia): A few drops of lavender oil in a diffuser for aromatherapy purposes.

For kids and adults:

8. Echinacea purpurea: For dose recommendations based on age, refer to the product's instructions or see a medical practitioner.

9. Panax ginseng: Adults should take 100–200 milligrams of ginseng daily. Consult with kids.

10. Adults should take 300–500 mg of Ashwagandha (Withania somnifera) per day. Consult with kids.

11. Milk Thistle (Silybum marianum): For dose recommendations based on age, refer to the product's instructions or see a medical expert.

12. Sacred Basil (Ocimum sanctum): Adults should take 300–600 mg daily. Consult with kids.

13. Adults should take 300–600 mg of nettle (Urtica dioica) daily. Consult with kids. 14. Moderate culinary usage of rosemary (Rosmarinus officinalis).

Regarding Adults:

15. 500–1,500 mg daily of Astragalus (Astragalus membranaceus).

16. 200–600 mg daily of licorice root (Glycyrrhiza glabra).

17. Foeniculum vulgare (fennel): Drink one to two cups of fennel tea daily.

18. Dandelion (Taraxacum officinale): Drink one to two cups of dandelion tea daily. 19. Sage (Salvia officinalis): Drink one to two cups of sage tea daily.

20. Origanum vulgare (oregano): moderate culinary usage.

Regarding Adults:

21. Thyme (Thymus vulgaris): Use sparingly in cooking.

22. Black Cohosh (Actaea racemosa): Read the directions on the packaging carefully or speak with a medical expert.

23. Valerian: 300–900 mg daily (Valeriana officinalis).

24. Ginkgo Biloba: Take 120–240 mg daily.

25. 300–600 mg daily of St. John's Wort (Hypericum perforatum).

26. Hawthorn (Crataegus monogyna): Refer to the directions on the packaging or a medical expert.

27. Saw Palmetto (Serenoa repens): Read the directions on the packaging carefully or speak with a medical expert.

28. Bilberry: 80–160 mg of bilberry extract daily (Vaccinium myrtillus).

Regarding Adults:

29. Even Primrose (Oenothera biennis): Read the directions on the packaging carefully, or get advice from a medical expert.

30. 500–1,000 mg daily of Passionflower (Passiflora incarnata).

Before beginning any herbal regimen, always see a specialist, especially if you have children, are pregnant, or have specific health issues. Individual reactions and dosages may differ.

Chapter 3: Benefits of Herbal Antibiotics

Exploring the Natural Healing Properties of Herbal Antibiotics

The potential for natural therapeutic effects of herbal antibiotics, which are derived from a variety of plants, has been acknowledged. Renowned for its capacity to strengthen the immune system, echinacea includes substances that encourage the formation of white blood cells, which strengthen the body's defense against illnesses. Another potent plant is garlic, which has broad-spectrum antimicrobial, antiviral, and antifungal effects because of its active ingredient, allicin. Berberine, found in goldenseal, is highly valued for its antibacterial properties, especially against bacteria and fungus. Turmeric has long been used medicinally because of its strong anti-inflammatory and antibacterial qualities, which are attributed to its active ingredient, curcumin. Carvacrol-rich oregano oil has potent antibacterial properties. Research indicates that it works well against a variety of bacteria, including types that are resistant to antibiotics. Similar antibacterial qualities are shown by thyme, which contains thymol and is hence a useful plant for treating infections. As an alternative to synthetic medicines, which might cause antibiotic resistance, these natural remedies are frequently helpful. Herbal medicines should be used cautiously, nevertheless, taking into account specific medical problems and any drug combinations. It is best to speak with a healthcare provider before adding herbal antibiotics to one's prescription. To sum up, herbal antibiotics provide a wide spectrum of all-natural therapeutic benefits, treating infections and enhancing general health. Combining these herbs with a healthy lifestyle may help keep the immune system strong and enhance the body's defenses against different infections.

Reducing side effects compared to pharmaceuticals

Joan and Dr. Marcus, two healers, worked in a little community tucked between undulating hills. Joan, a herbal antibiotic practitioner, trusted the efficacy of natural cures. Conversely, Dr. Marcus recommended pharmaceutical medications that were manufactured in clean labs. A mystery illness that affected several people in the community one day. Joan developed a mixture of herbal antibiotics by distilling strong ingredients from nearby plants.

Although the treatment worked well, some people had some stomach pain. While this was going on, Dr. Marcus administered a medication that quickly reduced symptoms, although some people had headaches and vertigo. Talks concerning the adverse impacts started as the village healed. Though softer, Joan's herbal medicine caused slight upset stomach symptoms. Despite certain side effects, Dr. Marcus praised the pharmacological treatment, highlighting its quick alleviation. The community encountered additional difficulties throughout time. Joan kept making improvements to her herbal antibiotics while taking community comments into consideration. Dr. Marcus also adjusted, looking for cutting-edge drug combinations to reduce adverse effects. Ultimately, the peasants acknowledged the benefits of both therapeutic approaches. Dr. Marcus's pharmaceutical medications provide quick relief but come with the danger of transient discomfort; Joan's herbal cures provide a natural option with fewer rapid side effects. In their hamlet, the healers created a holistic approach to treatment by combining scientific knowledge with the wisdom of nature.

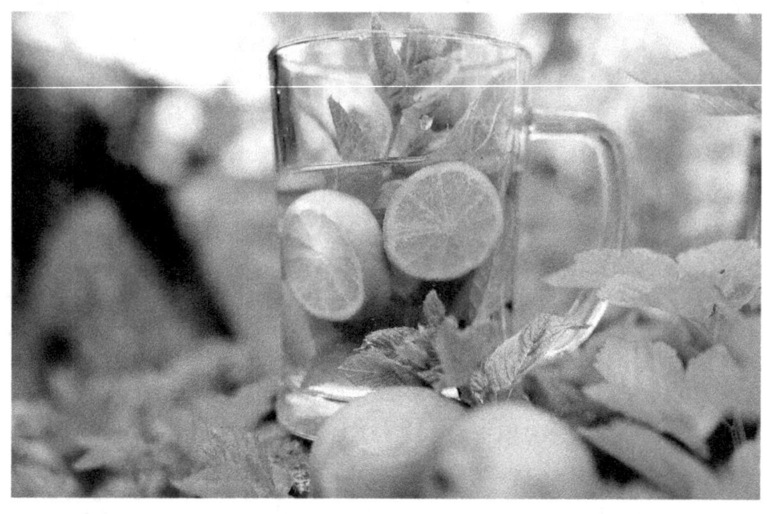

Supporting overall well-being

Herbal antibiotics are made from a variety of plants and other natural sources and offer a comprehensive approach to health that promotes general well-being. These natural substitutes are thought to strengthen the immune system, encourage bodily equilibrium, and provide possible advantages without the negative consequences linked to synthetic antibiotics. First of all, bioactive substances with antibacterial activities are frequently abundant in herbal antibiotics. For their antibacterial, antiviral, and antifungal qualities, ingredients including garlic, echinacea, and oregano have long been employed. These compounds could help fight infections and stop the emergence of bacterial strains that are resistant to treatment. Furthermore, it's believed that herbal antibiotics include anti-inflammatory properties that help lessen inflammation in the body. Herbal antibiotics may help to promote a more robust and balanced immune system by tackling chronic inflammation, which has been connected to a number of health problems. Furthermore, it is thought that a lot of herbal antibiotics aid in the body's natural detoxifying processes. Herbs like burdock and dandelion, for example, are often linked to liver health because they aid in the body's detoxification and the preservation of ideal organ function. Because the liver is essential to metabolism and the elimination of toxins, its health is directly related to general well-being. Moreover, there's a strong correlation between supporting gut health and using natural antibiotics. Ginger, turmeric, and licorice root are among the ingredients that are thought to encourage a varied and well-balanced gut flora and have favorable effects on the digestive system. Improved digestion, food absorption, and even mental health are linked to a healthy gut microbiota. A holistic approach to health that emphasizes immunological support, anti-inflammatory effects, detoxification, and gut health is in line with the potential advantages of herbal antibiotics, even if further study is necessary to fully understand their processes and efficacy. Including these natural cures in a balanced lifestyle might improve someone's general health.

Chapter 4: Incorporating Herbal Antibiotics into Daily Life

Integrating Herbal Antibiotics into Diet

Including natural plant-based medicines with antibacterial qualities in your diet is a way to include herbal antibiotics in your diet. Certain herbs have antibiotic-like properties and can be added to your meals to boost general health, but they should never be used in place of expert medical guidance.

1. Garlic: Toss in some fresh garlic when making stir-fries, spaghetti, or salads. Prepare garlic olive oil to drizzle over food or use in cooking.

2. Turmeric: Add powdered turmeric to stews, curries, and soups. Mix warm milk and turmeric to make a golden milk drink.

3. Oregano: Add dried oregano to salads, pizzas, and roasted veggies. Use olive oil infused with oregano as a dressing.

4. Thyme: Add freshly chopped thyme to vegetable or meat marinades. Steep dried or fresh thyme in boiling water to make thyme tea.

5. Echinacea: Use echinacea extract or tea to create a smoothie that strengthens the immune system. Incorporate echinacea into fruit-infused water or homemade popsicles.

6. Ginger: You may use grated ginger in smoothies, soups, and stir-fries. Boil fresh ginger slices in water to make ginger tea.

7. Manuka Honey: You may add manuka honey to yogurt or spread it on toast. To make a calming beverage, combine it with lemon in hot water.

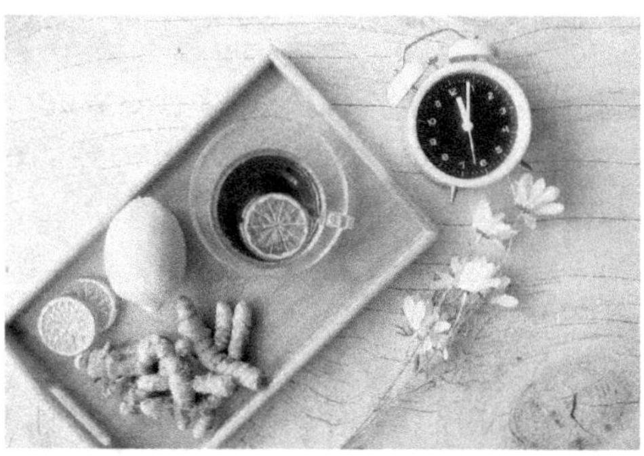

Always remember that moderation is vital and that you should always get medical advice before making major dietary changes. These herbal medicines can enhance overall health and be used in conjunction with a well-balanced diet. For individualized advice on managing a particular health issue, see a licensed healthcare professional.

Creating Herbal Remedies

Herbal medicine creation is a sophisticated procedure that combines scientific expertise with traditional wisdom. Start by doing an extensive study on herbs, looking at both modern scientific findings and their historical use. Understand that anecdotal evidence is not always trustworthy and give information from dependable sources—such as peer-reviewed research, herbalists, and reliable literature—priority. Experimentation with caution is necessary. Recognize the unique qualities of each plant, taking into account elements such as potency, possible adverse effects, and interactions with other drugs. Achieving the intended results while lowering dangers requires a precise and consistent dose. Harvesting methods that uphold ethics are crucial. Sustainable sourcing promotes ecological equilibrium and guarantees the long-term supply of therapeutic plants. To keep ecosystems intact, cultivate herbs responsibly or purchase them from reliable sources. It's critical to recognize that not all herbal medicines are secure or helpful for everyone. Individual reactions might differ, and certain herbs can have negative interactions with specific drugs or medical conditions. To ensure a thorough and knowledgeable approach to creating herbal remedies, get individual advice from qualified herbalists or medical specialists.

Lifestyle Practice for Optimal Well-being

Through the promotion of mental, emotional, and physical health, lifestyle choices are essential to reaching optimal wellness. These behaviors cover a wide range of topics, such as social interactions, stress management, sleep, physical exercise, and diet.

1. Diet: It is essential to have a balanced diet full of whole grains, fruits, vegetables, lean meats, and healthy fats. Maintaining enough hydration is crucial for maintaining both physical and general health. For instance, when making mealtime choices, go for natural foods rather than processed ones and include vibrant fruits and vegetables. For long-lasting energy, choose lean proteins like fish or lentils and include complete grains.

2. Activity Outside: Frequent exercise improves mood, helps control weight, and is good for the heart. It might take the form of regular exercises like cycling or walking. For instance, try to get in at least 150 minutes a week of moderate-to-intense activity. This can be riding a bike, going on quick walks, or doing enjoyable things like dancing or swimming.

3. Hygiene of Sleep: Restorative sleep is necessary for both the body and the mind. Crucial habits include reducing screen time before bed, maintaining a pleasant sleep environment, and establishing a consistent sleep regimen. For instance, make sure you get 7–9 hours of sleep every night by setting your alarm for the same time every day. Establish a calming bedtime regimen that includes deep breathing exercises or reading.

4. Handling stress: Prolonged stress can be harmful to one's health. Resilience may be increased by implementing stress-reduction strategies like mindfulness, meditation, or hobbies. For instance, set aside ten minutes each day for meditation or mindfulness exercises. Take part in joyful activities, such as drawing, spending time outdoors, or listening to music.

5. Network Relations: Developing and preserving healthy connections helps one's mental health and offers emotional support. For instance, encourage social relationships by spending time with friends and family on a regular basis. To increase the size of your social network, join clubs or groups that have similar interests.

A holistic approach to wellbeing is created by incorporating various lifestyle behaviors that support mental clarity, emotional resilience, and physical health. An ideal and well-rounded lifestyle is built on the foundation of consistency in these practices.

Chapter 5: Safety and Precautions

Advising on proper usage

1. Speak with a medical expert: Before taking herbal antibiotics, always see a healthcare professional to be sure they are safe and suitable for your situation.

2. Herb research: Learn everything you can about the herbs you intend to employ. Some examples include oregano (Origanum vulgare), echinacea (Echinacea purpurea), and garlic (Allium sativum).

3. Know dosage: Take herbal antibiotics as prescribed; going beyond might have negative consequences. For example, due to possible adverse effects, the use of golden seal (Hydrastis canadensis) should be done with caution.

4. Take into account synergistic blends: Certain plants complement each other effectively. For instance, mixing sage (Salvia officinalis) and thyme (Thymus vulgaris) may strengthen their antibacterial qualities.

5. Rotate herbs: Alternate herbal antibiotics to avoid resistance. It might be helpful to alternate

between alternatives like oregano and herbs that contain berberine.

6. Quality matters. Use fresh herbs or select premium herbal supplements. For instance, allicin, a strong antibacterial substance, is frequently present in premium garlic supplements.

7. Exercise patience: Results from herbal antibiotics might not happen right away. Allow enough time for them to work before anticipating prompt relief.

8. Take herbal teas into consideration: Add herbs to teas for a calming and efficient delivery system. For example, ginger tea contains antibacterial and anti-inflammatory qualities.

9. Maintain a healthy diet: While using herbal antibiotics, strengthen your immune system by eating a balanced diet. The benefits of turmeric (Curcuma longa) include immunological stimulation and anti-inflammatory effects.

10. Drink plenty of water. Drinking enough water aids in the body's toxin removal process. For best outcomes, take herbal treatments in conjunction with enough water consumption.

11. Incorporate probiotics:To preserve a healthy balance of gut flora while using herbal

antibiotics, include meals high in probiotics, such as yogurt.

12. Keep an eye out for allergies. Recognize that herbs may cause allergic responses. For example, chamomile (Matricaria chamomilla) allergy sufferers may also experience adverse effects from ragweed.

13. Steer clear of this when pregnant: It might not be safe to use some natural antibiotics while pregnant. Before using it, speak with your doctor and think about using alternatives, such as honey, to relieve sore throats.

14. Watch for side effects: Be mindful of any unfavorable responses. For instance, using Melaleuca alternifolia (tea tree) oil excessively might irritate the skin.

15. Incorporate with traditional medical care: antibiotics derived from plants can support medical therapies. Talk to your doctor about any possible interactions.

16. Store properly. Keep herbal antibiotics potent by keeping them out of direct sunlight and in a cool, dry environment.

17. Maintain consistency: For best results, stick to a regular schedule. For example, regular consumption of astragalus (Astragalus

membranaceus) may enhance immunological function.

18. Take into account the underlying cause: Take care of the problem that is causing the infection or sickness. Antibiotics made from herbs can be used in a comprehensive health program.

19. Educate others: disseminate your expertise in a responsible manner, stressing the need to speak with medical specialists before using herbal antibiotics as self-medication.

20. Listen to your body: Be mindful of how herbal antibiotics affect your body's response and modify your strategy accordingly. Consult a medical professional if symptoms worsen.

Potential Interaction with Medication

Herbs and pharmaceuticals can interact in complicated ways, so use caution when doing so. For example, St. John's Wort may interfere with blood thinners and antidepressants, changing how well they work. Likewise, supplements containing garlic may intensify the anticoagulant effects of blood thinners, which may result in bleeding problems. Renowned for its cognitive advantages, ginkgo biloba may worsen bleeding risks and conflict with blood clotting drugs. In the meantime, the well-known herb echinacea may have an impact on immunosuppressant medication metabolism, hence decreasing its effectiveness. Because of its hepatoprotective qualities, it is important to take into account the possible effect on liver function while taking certain drugs with herbs like milk thistle. On the other hand, grapefruit juice has the ability to suppress the enzymes in charge of drug metabolism, which can impact the absorption of certain drugs and result in quantities in the circulation that aren't expected. To minimize such interactions, patients should be transparent with their healthcare professionals about their use of herbs. Medical practitioners may offer tailored guidance based on specific medical problems and prescription schedules, guaranteeing a comprehensive approach to wellbeing and reducing the possibility of herb-drug interactions. To maintain ideal health results, treatment programs may need to be modified and monitored on a regular basis.

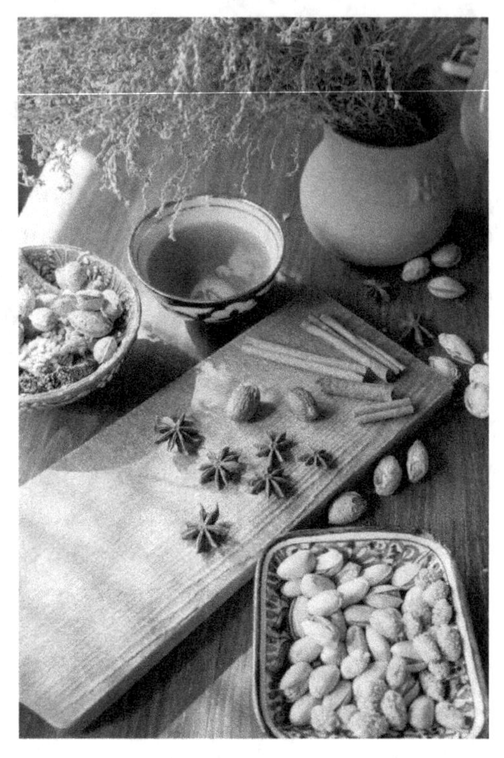

Chapter 6: Building Your Herbal Medicine Kit

Essential herbs to have on hand

Lavender: Reason: Lavender is a necessary ingredient for establishing a peaceful atmosphere because of its well-known calming effects. It can help promote better sleep and lessen worry and tension.

Peppermint: Reason: Peppermint has several uses and can be used to treat headaches, nausea, and indigestion. Its energizing scent can also aid in easing mental exhaustion.

Aloe vera: Aloe vera is prized for its therapeutic qualities and is a home cure for wounds, burns, and skin irritations. When used topically, it has calming and restorative properties.

Chamomile: The well-known sedative properties of chamomile make it a great tea option for fostering calmness and improved sleep. It has anti-inflammatory qualities as well.

Rosemary: Reason: In addition to its culinary use, rosemary is recognized for enhancing focus and recall. It may be used in a variety of recipes and provides a revitalizing scent to the surrounding area.

Echinacea: Echinacea is beneficial for preventing and treating cold and flu symptoms because of its immune-boosting qualities. It aids the body's built-in defensive systems.

Ginger: Reason: Ginger is an effective treatment for inflammation, dyspepsia, and nausea. It may be used in meals or as a calming ginger tea; it's quite flexible.

Turmeric: Reason: A mainstay of herbal therapy, turmeric is well-known for its anti-inflammatory and antioxidant qualities. It has several health advantages and may be used as a supplement or in cooking.

Reason: Mint relieves indigestion and bloating and is a great remedy for digestive problems. It may be used as a garnish or used in teas; it's very refreshing.

Thyme: Reason: Thyme is good for respiratory health because of its antibacterial qualities. It helps strengthen the immune system and may be added to drinks or food recipes.

These foundational herbs support mental and emotional equilibrium in addition to physical health, forming a holistic approach to health.

Storage and shelf life considerations

Herbal antibiotics must be stored properly to preserve their efficacy and security. Here are some common storage recommendations for natural antibiotics:

1. Cool, dark area: Keep herbal antibiotics out of direct sunlight and in a cool, dark area. Herbal components might lose some of their efficacy when exposed to heat and light.

2. Airtight Containers: To keep herbs dry and protected from the elements, use airtight containers. Hermetic sealing aids in preserving the quality of the herbs by preventing oxidation.

3. Dry Environment: Make sure the area where herbal antibiotics are kept is dry. Moisture can encourage the formation of mold and lessen the medicinal effects of the plants.

4. Glass or dark-colored containers: To avoid interactions with plastic, keep herbs in glass containers wherever feasible. Dark-colored glass offers further protection by helping to filter out light.

5. Labeling and Date: Write the herb's name, its intended use, and the date of purchase or

preparation clearly on each container. This guarantees that you can quickly determine and monitor the herbal antibiotics' freshness.

6. Herbs That Benefit from Refrigeration: Some herbs could be better off being refrigerated. Verify the particular advice given for the herbs you are keeping. For instance, it's usually safest to store oils or tinctures steeped in garlic in the refrigerator.

7. Safe, Childproof Storage: To avoid unintentional consumption if you have kids, make sure herbal antibiotics are kept in a safe, childproof area.

8. Regular Inspection: Check your herbal antibiotics from time to time for any indications of mold, discoloration, or strange smells.

Throw out the herbs if you see any changes. Keep in mind that the type of plant used and its preparation might affect how long herbal antibiotics last on the market. It is always advisable to heed any particular storage advice given by manufacturers or herbalists. When in doubt, get individualized guidance from a herbalist or medical expert.

DIY Herbal Medicine Recipes

Making your own herbal remedies at home may be a fulfilling and healthy approach to dealing with a range of health issues. Here are some basic recipes for herbal medicines and their intended uses:

1. Recipe: Ginger-Honey Syrup Ingredients: fresh ginger, honey. Grate some fresh ginger and add some honey to it. Give it a few hours, or perhaps overnight, to sit. To relieve sore throats and aid with digestion, take one teaspoon.

2. Calendula Salve: Ingredients: beeswax, olive oil, or carrier oil. * Recipe: Pour oil over dried calendula flowers, drain, and then stir in melted beeswax. Transfer it to a container. Applying calendula salve topically can aid in the healing of damaged skin.

3. Elderberry Syrup:Ingredients: water, honey, and dried elderberries. Recipe: Bring water to a simmer, add dried elderberries, drain, and stir in honey. Because of its reputation for enhancing immunity, elderberry syrup is frequently taken throughout the cold and flu season.

4. Sweet Theatre: Contents: dried peppermint leaves. How to Make It: In boiling water, steep

dried peppermint leaves. In addition to being a generally calming beverage, peppermint tea works wonders for headaches and stomach problems.

5. Lavender and Chamomile Sleep Tincture: Containings: alcohol, dried lavender, and dried chamomile flowers. Instructions: Put the dried lavender and chamomile flowers in a container, pour alcohol over the top, and let it sit for a few weeks. To encourage relaxation and facilitate sleep, strain and use a few drops.

6. Olive Oil and Garlic Infusion: Ingredients: olive oil and garlic cloves. Recipe: For a few weeks, crush the garlic cloves and let them marinate in olive oil. Use the oil topically to benefit from its antibacterial qualities after straining.

7. Golden Milk Paste: Contents: coconut oil, black pepper, and turmeric powder. Instructions: To make a paste, combine turmeric, coconut oil, and black pepper. This makes a soothing and anti-inflammatory golden milk beverage when added to heated milk.

Do your homework on the characteristics and possible side effects of each plant, and seek medical advice if you are on medication or have any health issues.

Conclusion

Many people are looking into the field of herbal antibiotics as a potential answer in light of the growing antibiotic resistance in the world. Herbal antibiotics, which harness the force of nature, are a strong substitute for synthetic medications and offer a comprehensive approach to health and wellness. Herbal antibiotics come from a variety of plants, each of which has special qualities that have been known to have therapeutic use for ages. Natural medicines such as garlic, which has strong antimicrobial qualities, and oregano oil, which has antibacterial and antifungal effects, have been used in traditional medicine for generations. Using herbal antibiotics is about more than simply finding a substitute; it's also about reestablishing a connection with nature's pharmacy and drawing on the knowledge that has been accumulated over many centuries. Many herbs provide additional health advantages, such as antioxidant and anti-inflammatory qualities, in addition to their antibacterial activities. This all-encompassing method of treatment takes into account the underlying physiological imbalances as well as the symptoms. Setting the priority of natural treatments for yourself is a deliberate decision to begin your road towards maximum wellbeing with herbal antibiotics. It's about realizing that nature offers us a variety of resources to enhance our well-being and that health is a dynamic equilibrium. By including these herbs in our regular routines, we may take a proactive approach to prevention and foster resilience in the face of frequent illnesses. Adopting herbal antibiotics as a component of an all-encompassing wellness plan is the call to action. Begin by adding these herbs to your diet, either as supplements or in your cooking. Incorporate therapeutic techniques such as tinctures and herbal teas into your everyday routine to get the benefits. To create a strategy that suits your specific needs, think about speaking with a licensed herbalist or medical expert. Reaching optimal well-being is a process, not a finish line. Adopting herbal medications is a way to support the larger fight against antibiotic resistance in addition to investing in your own health. It's an exhortation to nurture a sustainable attitude toward wellbeing, get back in touch with nature, and pay attention to your body. As you set out on your herbal wellness journey, keep in mind that gradual, steady progress produces significant results. Accept the healing properties of herbal antibiotics and let the natural world lead you to enduring health and vigor.

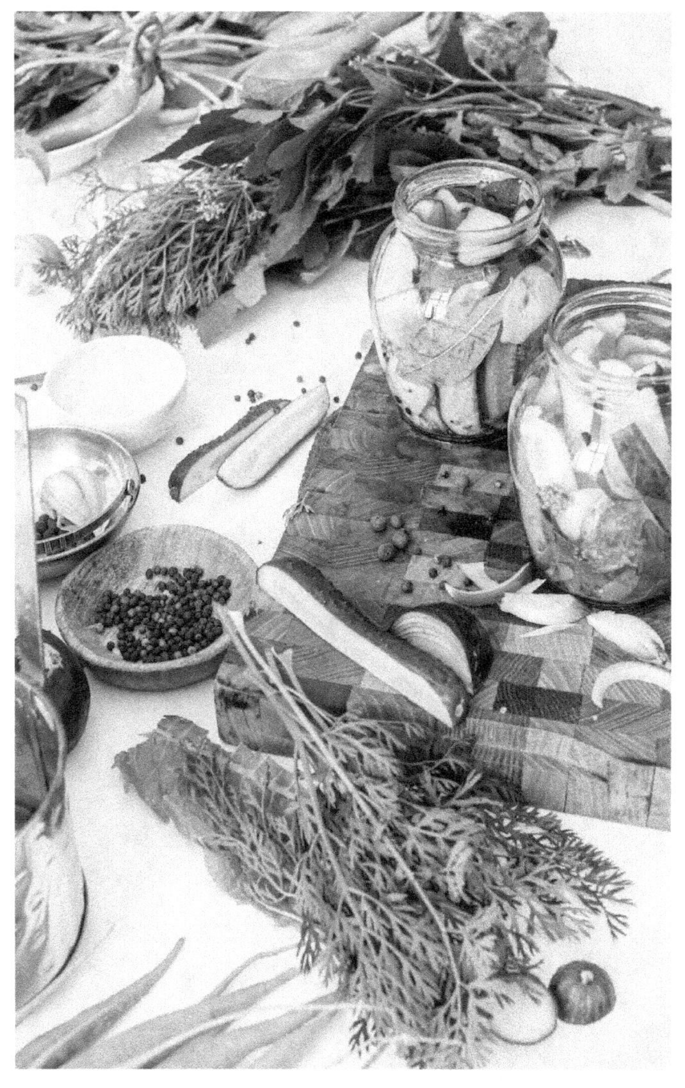